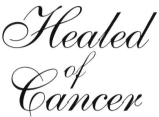

Healed of Cancer

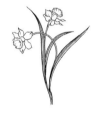

by Dodie Osteen

Healed of Cancer
Dodie Osteen

Unless otherwise indicated, all Scripture quotations in this book are
from the New King James Version of the Bible / Thomas Nelson
Publishers, Nashville: Thomas Nelson Publishers.,
Copyright © 1982. Used by permission. All rights reserved.

Scripture quotations marked "TLB" or "The Living Bible" are
taken from The Living Bible Kenneth N. Taylor. Wheaton: Tyndale
House, 1997, © 1971 by Tyndale House Publishers, Inc. Used by
permission. All rights reserved.

For a list of available books by John Osteen write to:
Lakewood Church
P.O. Box 23297
Houston, TX 77228
Customer Service 1-800-278-0520

ISBN 0-912631-33-3

Contents

Healed of Cancer

I am so thankful to be alive today and to be able to bring you a message of hope! That is what Jesus is, Hope. I feel like the Psalmist David who said, *O Lord…I pleaded with you, and you gave me my health again. You brought me back from the brink of the grave, from death itself, and here I am alive!* (Psalm 30:2-3, TLB).

The Word of God is extremely important to people who are fighting a battle with their health, because it's sometime the only hope they have. I know I would have died if it had not been for the Bible. For many years, I had been taught the truth from God's Word. I had heard faith messages that built me up. I knew that Jesus didn't want His children sick and that He not only died for our sins but also for our sicknesses. If it were not for the Word of God, I would not be alive and writing this book.

God said, *My people are destroyed for lack of knowledge* (Hosea 4:6). This is a sad thing, but it's true. Many people do not know that it is God's will for them to be healed. And this information is the difference between life and death!

In another psalm, David said, *How we thank you, Lord! Your mighty miracles give proof that you care* (Psalm 75:1, TLB).

God does care for His children. The fact that He healed me shows me He cares, and that He wants to heal you, too.

Hebrews 11:1 says, *Now faith is the substance of things HOPED for* (emphasis mine). If you have cancer, a kidney disorder, or some other terminal disease that has brought pain and sickness in your body, I want you to know there is hope in Jesus. He does not want you to die an early death. He wants you to live and declare the works of the Lord (see Psalm 118:17).

I've Always Been Healthy and Active

I have always worked hard and stayed busy all the time. I like to work. I have always enjoyed working. Our children say, "We have never seen our mother idle. She works all the time." John used to say, "Dodie, it's time for you to stop working now. You've done enough for today."

I have always been healthy. Thank God! I had polio when I was a baby, but I don't remember that. I don't believe during all our married life that John had seen me sick in bed unless I was recuperating from the birth of one of our children. So I was used to excellent health. I was thankful for good health, but I realize now that maybe I took it for granted.

I remember, when somebody would ask, "How are you?" I would reply, "I am disgustingly healthy!" After I was diagnosed with cancer, I realized how foolish those words were.

My days now are precious to me. I thought they would always be there. I learned not to say idle words. Thank God for your health, and be grateful for every day of life He gives you.

How It All Started

In October 1981, symptoms began to appear in my body. It was at a time when my husband and I had so much going for us. Our children were getting older and I was freer than I had been in years. Our youngest child was sixteen years old. I had many plans for the future.

John and I had been invited to be special guests for the opening of the Oral Roberts City of Faith Medical and Research Center in Tulsa, Oklahoma. Our son Paul was a student at the Oral Roberts Medical School at the time, so we were thrilled about being a part of that great celebration.

During the first day, John and I had a wonderful time together, but that night I began to experience symptoms of illness. I felt a bit fuzzy in my mind, and I had chills and a fever. I would be freezing cold, yet burning up with fever. These symptoms got progressively worse for the next three weeks. I was unable to sleep, and when you lose sleep over a long period of time, it does something to you. I became extremely weak. After a few weeks, I became jaundiced and other symptoms and pains began to appear.

During this time, I kept trying to do my housework and take part in all the church services. I especially remember a service when I was so weak that I couldn't get up. I had knelt down to pray for a lady and when I started to get up, I discovered I couldn't. I had to crawl over to a chair to pull myself up. Nobody knew then, not even me, how sick I really was.

John and I believed and confessed God's Word. We sought God and agreed together in prayer. I was anointed with oil according to James 5:14-15. I did everything I knew to do. But I got worse.

At the time all this was happening to me, our big Thanksgiving convention at Lakewood Church was coming up, and many plans were being made for that event. I had already bought some new clothes and I was really excited. John and I decided that I should see a doctor and get some help so that I would be well and strong to participate fully.

We called the City of Faith and they recommended a doctor in our own city of Houston. At that time, the City of Faith was not capable of handling too many patients or I would have gone there. That would have been my first choice. However, they had just opened and did not have their facilities up to full capacity yet. I took their counsel and saw a local physician, a wonderful Christian whose specialty is internal medicine.

After examining me, he said, "Mrs. Osteen, I think you should go into the hospital for some tests."

I said, "May I go in as an outpatient? We have a big convention coming up next week."

He said, "No, I think you will need to have more extensive tests than that."

I consented to go in the hospital, thinking I would be there for only two or three days. It turned out to be twenty. I had just about every kind of test there is: several sonograms, two C.T. scans, an upper and lower G.I. series, a bone marrow biopsy, and a uterine biopsy. You name it, I had it!

The doctors' first diagnosis was that I had a liver abscess, probably caused from some germ picked up on one of our mission trips to India. They treated me with a medication which had many side effects, but which they hoped would clear up the abscess.

Some of the side effects were nausea and depression. Just being in the hospital was depressing to me, there was so much oppression there. The medicine also made my mind fuzzy and I was unable to think clearly. I became terribly tired and weak. I could hardly get out of bed.

Further tests revealed no destructive bacteria, amoebae, or parasites. This, consequently, confounded the first diagnosis, and more sophisticated tests were ordered.

Finally, one day the doctor came into my room and said, "I have sent some blood work to Cincinnati."

"Why would you do that?" I asked. "There are plenty of excellent hospitals here in Houston."

He replied, "This is just for my own peace of mind. But I feel sure there is no malignancy in your body."

Cancer,
The Sentence of Death!

Malignancy!

I was astounded by that word! Up to this time, the possibility of cancer had never entered my mind. For years I had confessed that I would never have cancer or any other disease. When he said that, I thought, *This is not what I expected at all. I don't want the word cancer ever mentioned in my room again.*

I called John on the telephone and told him what the doctor had said. "I don't want you to say the word cancer," I said, "because I don't have cancer. *I will not* have cancer!"

On Thursday, December 10, John came to the hospital to visit me. The doctor met him in the lobby with devastating news. He said, "Pastor, your wife has metastatic cancer of the liver. With or without chemotherapy, she has only a few weeks to live. We can treat her, but it will only slightly prolong her life.

"However, we cannot find the primary tumor," he said. "We don't know where it is. In fact, it has really baffled us. Usually a primary tumor signifies the beginning of cancer and then it spreads to the

11

liver or kidneys or some other organ. But we cannot find one. With your consent, we would like to do exploratory surgery or a colonoscopy to try to locate the tumor."

John couldn't believe it. He said, "Doctor, I am going to take my wife home. We are going to pray and seek God, and then we will decide what to do. We believe in miracles, and we believe in the Miracle Worker."

The doctor said, "Well, Pastor, you're going to have to have a miracle this time."

When John told me the diagnosis, I was surprised at myself. I was stunned and shocked, but there was no hysteria. I just sat quietly and listened. The doctor came in soon afterwards and we talked.

One thing did upset me, however. Our son Paul, now a medical intern, happened to be doing surgery at Hermann Hospital in Houston, just down the street from the hospital where I was. John called him and said, "Son, come over to the hospital. Mother needs you." He ran all the way!

Soon I heard this tremendous sobbing out in the hallway. I didn't know who it was at first. Then I recognized that it was my first born son, Paul.

Paul had watched me during the first weeks of my sickness, and he was very concerned. Being a medical doctor, he knew the prognosis of a person diagnosed with liver cancer, and it tore him up. Paul knew God could heal, but he had been trained medically to know that a person dies with cancer of the liver. There is usually not much hope.

When Paul came in my room, I said, "Son, we have a battle on our hands. You are going to have to be a fighter with me now."

He said, "Okay, Mother." He regained his composure, and he was strong with me throughout the battle.

All my family was supportive and optimistic. I am an only child, and my parents, even though they were elderly, never panicked. They stood strong, like the pillars of strength they have always been. When they heard I was being released from the hospital they were there at the house, ready to care for me and the family.

I Went Home

I went home on December 10, 1981, and I never did go back to the hospital. However, my advice is, if you have cancer and you can be helped by chemotherapy, by all means take it if you feel you should. Do whatever you feel peace about in your heart.

I do not advise anyone to do what I did just because it worked for me. The doctors gave me only a few weeks to live with or without chemotherapy, and I chose not to have it. But God leads and directs each of us individually. This is the way He led me in my faith.

My Faith Had To Take Over Now

While I was in the hospital, I was so weak, and my senses were so dulled by medication, that I depended heavily on other people's prayers and faith.

I received phone calls from Oral Roberts and Kenneth Hagin. I had calls from Kenneth Copeland and Daisy and T. L. Osborn. Daisy even came to visit me at the hospital. Most of all, I depended on my husband. I was married 44 years to a great teacher of the Word of God, and he constantly encouraged me and spoke the Word of God to me. I also relied on the people of Lakewood Church who were praying and fasting for me. Other people's prayers had to "carry" me during this time.

It was soon after I came home, however, that I realized my healing was a personal matter between me and Jesus.

One night, in the early hours of the morning,

God spoke to my heart: "It is not your husband's faith; it is not Oral Roberts' faith; it is not Kenneth Hagin's faith; it is YOUR faith that you must go on now." I knew it was between me and Jesus from that time on.

This was a different situation than when our daughter Lisa was born with cerebral palsy. (An account of Lisa's miracle is told in *There Is a Miracle in Your Mouth,* by John Osteen.) Lisa is grown and perfectly normal now. John and I both believed God for her healing even though we did not have much knowledge of the Word of God then. She was a baby and, of course, unable to believe God for herself. She was healed by our faith in God and His great mercy.

The Fight of Faith

Once I arrived home, I never did go to bed to be cared for by others. I felt that if I did, it would demonstrate unbelief and undermine my faith. I went to bed only at night during normal sleeping hours. I wouldn't even take a nap. I knew if I did, I would stay there because I felt so sick.

My first morning home I got up, bathed, and put on a dress that now swallowed my 89-pound frame. I was not going to act sick.

Healed of Cancer

John and I believed in the power of the prayer of agreement. Jesus said, *If two of you agree on earth concerning anything that they ask, it will be done for them by My Father in heaven* (Matthew 18:19).

The day after I came home from the hospital, I asked John to pray with me. I said, "Darling, you are the head of this house. You are going to have to take authority over this cancer in my body. We must agree that God is going to heal me and make me whole."

So we did. John anointed me with oil as we both got on the floor in our bedroom, face down before God, and he took authority over any disease and over any cancerous cells in my body.

That was December 11, 1981. As far as I'm concerned, that's the day my healing began. I had the confidence in God's Word that I was healed. But my body did not completely line up with that truth. I still had many symptoms, and I still felt ill, but in my heart I knew I was healed!

It took a long time for the symptoms to go. Many times I felt like saying, "Jesus, it would be so much easier just to give up the fight and go on to be with You." Instead, though, I had to fight. I read Isaiah 43:25, 26, which says, *I, even I, am He who blots out your transgressions for my own*

16

sake; and I will not remember your sins. Put me in remembrance; let us contend together; state your case, that you may be acquitted.

In the middle of the night, when everybody else was asleep, I pled my case with Jesus. I said, "Jesus, I don't want to die. I am too young to die. You said that we can choose life or death, and I don't choose to die. I will not die, but live and declare the works of the Lord" (see Psalm 118:17).

I reminded the Lord that my husband needed me, my children needed me, my flock needed me, my mother and daddy needed me, and HE needed me.

I examined my heart, and God began to deal with me about some things. One night I wrote letters to seven people whom I felt I might have offended, whom I needed to forgive or who needed to forgive me. I even wrote letters to people I thought I might have offended after I became sick because I had been so irritable. I hadn't been myself. One letter was to my husband; others were for each of my children and a pastor that I felt I spoke to sharply.

I did everything I knew to do that would help me have a positive, hopeful attitude. I placed a picture of me in my wedding dress by my bed. I would pray, Oh, Lord, if I could just feel like I did on my wedding day! I also put out a picture of me riding a horse when we were vacationing at a ranch. I was the picture of health. I thought, *Oh, God, if I could just ride a horse again!*

Another thing that was good for me was going out and praying for others. James 5:16 says, *Pray for one another, that you may be healed*. When you are fighting a battle, if you will give out of your need, God will cause your answer to come to you quicker. Luke 6:38 says, *Give, and it will be given to you*. When you get your mind so much on yourself and your own need, you begin to weaken.

I was so sick that I did not feel like going out. When I was in the house alone, I thought about myself, the pain, sickness, and symptoms, and I would get weary and full of pity. But when I forced myself to go out and pray for someone else, my health began to come back to me. I remember one time I drove across town a long way from our house to pray for somebody in the hospital. After visiting that person, God impressed me to go by another home where the man had been sick a long time. I was so tired! I did not feel like going at all, but I went. I almost dropped from exhaustion. The point is that I felt in my own heart that I had been obedient to God.

The Word Became
My Life

In spite of every discouraging symptom, my heart knew that God's Word could not lie. I had confidence in God's Word. If I hadn't, I would have died. Hebrews 10:23 says, *Let us hold fast the confession of our hope without wavering, for He who promised is faithful.*

Day by day, I gained hope and encouragement from the precious promises that God revealed to me through His Word. I clung to my Bible and its healing promises. The Word became my life. I read and confessed the Scriptures daily.

There were days, however, when I wavered in my faith, and I would feel great condemnation. My confession of faith had not changed, but it seemed like I was wavering. I think anybody who fights a long battle with sickness will waver some if symptoms persist.

It wasn't until I talked this over with my husband that I realized the wavering was in my head, not my heart. I said, "John, what is wrong with me? I feel so condemned because I am wavering."

John knew just what to say. He asked, "Dodie,

are you wavering in your heart?"

I said, "No. I know God's Word wouldn't lie to me. It's true."

"Then where are you wavering?"

I considered his question, then replied, "In my head!"

"Well," John said, "don't you see? That's the difference. You are not wavering in your heart, because you know God's Word is true. There is no need for you to be condemned. Your heart is established. Resist the thoughts from the devil, and he will flee from you."

That helped me so much! I had confidence in my heart, but the devil was using my thoughts to cause me to doubt. I had faith in my heart, but doubt in my mind.

If you are having symptoms of your sickness and you seem to be wavering, check your spirit.

You are probably not wavering in your heart. Doubt is from your head. Don't let the devil condemn you.

How I Fought Fear

People often ask me if I struggled with fear. Oh, how I battled with fear! When I was strong in my body, I never felt fear, but when I was weak and sick, fear would overwhelm me.

I want to be honest with you. I am the wife of a pastor and faith teacher, but first of all, I am a human being. I have thoughts and feelings just like anyone else. I had to cast down imaginations. I laughed at symptoms.

I am a registered nurse. I understood how my body was supposed to function, and I understood that it wasn't functioning properly. Certain things the doctors had said now brought fear to my heart. Those were the thoughts I had to fight against most, and I still have to resist them sometimes.

Satan would torment me with the doctor's words, "You have only a few weeks to live. . . few weeks to live. . .few weeks to live." He would use pain and then say, "You're going to die. Have your family bury you in that pretty pink dress. You look good in it."

But I would replace those thoughts with God's Word and say, "With long life will He satisfy me, and show me His salvation" (see Psalm 91:16). The devil bombarded my mind with every kind of fear imaginable, especially when everybody was asleep and I lay awake. Symptoms came against my body, mostly demonic and tormenting thoughts, just to try my faith.

I fought so hard in the middle of the night! This

is when the devil's thoughts would play on my mind. Many nights I would lie awake and pray continually and rebuke the spirit of fear. I felt like I had battle fatigue, but I kept on pushing and fighting.

In order to keep my mind from drifting to the negative, I would walk around, saying with every step, "By the stripes of Jesus, I am healed. . .by the stripes of Jesus, I am healed" (see 1 Peter 2:24).

I would meditate on scriptures like, *It is God who works in you both to will and to do for His good pleasure* (Philippians 2:13).

The Word of God would always encourage me and make me feel better, but the devil challenged every step of faith I took. Each time I quoted Scripture, he would say, "It hasn't done you one bit of good to confess the Word of God, has it?" He would question every promise of God.

I quoted scripture after scripture. (See Chapter 2 for a list of the scriptures I used most.) Daily, as I used God's Word, I became stronger and stronger.

Is Tormenting Fear
Normal for a Christian?

I was once asked, "Is this fear a normal thing for

a Spirit-filled Christian?" I do not know what you consider normal. I am just telling you what I went through. Don't be critical of people unless you walk in their shoes. If you don't think they have as much faith as you do, don't be critical of them. Try to realize what they are going through. No matter how much you know, you still do not know all they are facing. I have been critical of others in the past. I am ashamed because now I know what I went through.

God Did Not Give Me Cancer

Did God send this sickness on me?

No, of course not. Both my heart and my mind knew it was not God's will for me or any of His children to be sick.

If I'd had any doubt in my mind about it being God's will for me to be well, I would never have gotten well. That is why we need to fight the lies of the devil. That is why we need to teach people God's Word. Get it clearly established in your mind and heart that it IS God's will for you to be well.

God did not put cancer on me. Jesus said it was "the thief," Satan, who came to steal my health, kill me, and destroy me. Jesus said, *I am come that*

[you] *might have life, and that* [you] *might have it more abundantly* (John 10:10, KJV). Notice, that verse says that you "might" have life. You have a choice. You do not have to have abundant life, but you CAN if you want to. I wanted to, so I pled my case with God.

People Everywhere Prayed For Me

Everyone was so good! I wasn't physically able to travel anywhere to have people pray for me. I asked God to send people to pray for me in my own home. And they began to come.

Many people came from great distances. I remember one lady flew to Houston from across the nation to pray for me and tell me how God had healed her of cancer. Our entire church stood with us and interceded. They helped us in innumerable ways. Everyone encouraged me, especially my family.

I want to encourage husbands and wives and children to stay close together, because you need each other, especially when a crisis comes. My husband and my children would say to me every day, "You are healed."

It means so much to have somebody close to you stand with you in prayer when you are fighting a disease. John stood with me and encouraged me. He saw me crying and hurting when nobody else knew it.

Some days I didn't feel like doing anything but cry. He would tell me over and over, "Sweetheart, you're going to get well. We are going to go all over the world together. We're going to do things for Jesus. You're a good soldier. Jesus has confidence in you. Our best days are ahead."

He would hold my hand and pray in the Spirit. He would seek God, and God would show him things in the Word which he would share with me. When my faith seemed to weaken, it would always be lifted by something John would say or by some special way the Lord would speak to my heart. John encouraged me and increased my faith in any and every way He could.

A Visitation
From The Lord

One day we had a special visitation from the Lord in our bedroom. I believe an angel actually came to strengthen us.

We had come home from a church service and John went to the bedroom to hang up his coat. He walked through the door and noticed his Bible open on the bed where he had left it earlier that day. As he turned around, he heard someone turning the pages of his Bible. There was no draft or wind coming into the room from any direction.

When he looked closely, a page was supernaturally turned under on one edge and Psalm 105:37 was quickened to him on that page. *He brought them forth also with silver and gold: and there was not one feeble person among their tribes* (KJV).

How we praised God for that word!

My Family Treated Me As If I Were Well

My children treated me as if I were a normal, healthy mother. From the time John and I prayed, they believed that I was healed. Sometimes there were things in the house that needed to be done, which I would ask them to do. But because they believed I was healed, they insisted that I could do them.

It is a good thing they treated me as if I were healed; otherwise, many times I would have been tempted to have pity parties. They would not allow me to feel sorry for myself. They reminded me of the Word of God and of the prayer of faith we had prayed.

One time I wanted a piece of furniture moved

to another place in the room. It was a small article that I normally could have moved. When I asked for help, one of them said, "Mother, you are healed. You can do it." And I could! It was difficult, but it made me use my faith. This irritated me then. But, to my children, I was healed. I thank God they have been grounded in the Word of God.

Don't sit around and feel sorry for yourself when you are fighting the battle for your healing. Pity never wins! I overcame my pity parties by speaking to my body and commanding it to come in line with the Word of God. And it did!

Confirming My Miracle

People are always asking me if I have been back to the doctor to confirm my healing. I once received a letter from a doctor's sister asking, "Has this healing been documented?"

If by "documentation" people mean did I go back to the same doctors and have the same tests run again, no, I haven't. However, over the years I have been examined by other doctors for other medical reasons, and they have confirmed my healing. (See Chapter 3.)

I never felt peace about going back to the hospital for tests to prove I was healed. You might think that is strange. But I didn't want anything disturbing my faith. I know that I am healed. I left the hospital December 10, 1981, and today I am still alive, full of energy, and very active many years longer than the few weeks the doctors gave me to live back in 1981. The fact that I am still living is a pretty good indication that the Word of God works!

Some time after I left the hospital, I decided to go to a gynecologist for a checkup. Only John and I know all the things that came against my body to try our faith. One of them was abnormal bleeding accompanied by severe pain in the abdomen. So I made an appointment with Dr. Richard W. Walker, Jr., a fine Christian gynecologist who attends Lakewood Church. He knew of my condition and what I'd been through.

Since the doctors at the hospital had not found a primary tumor, the devil had tormented me for months with the fear that I had a malignant cyst or tumor growing in my body. My former gynecologist had diagnosed a small fibroid tumor on the wall of my uterus several years before. These tumors are usually benign, and, because it was small, he recommended that nothing be done. However, the physicians in the hospital had suggested this might be the site of the primary

Healed of Cancer

tumor.

John and I prayed all the way to Dr. Richard Walker's office. His examination showed that indeed the fibroid tumor had grown. It was now the size of a golf ball, and he recommended a hysterectomy to remove my uterus.

I battled whether to have the surgery or not, but finally consented. Examination under anesthesia immediately before surgery revealed the golf ball-sized mass on the wall of my uterus. After surgery, when the pathologist ran the necessary tests for his report, no tumor could be found. It was a miracle! Today, Dr. Walker reports I am as healthy as a young woman!

Then in November 1983, a full two years after receiving my death sentence of cancer, I felt I should have some blood work done because my blood count had been so low in the hospital. I went to Dr. Reginald B. Cherry, a doctor of preventive medicine who was a member of our church at that time. He is a wonderful man, saved and filled with the Holy Spirit. He has always been an encourager and an uplifter to me.

The test results confirmed that God had performed a miracle! The blood work was normal. And seven liver function tests were completely normal. No cancer! Glory to God!

Jesus hasn't changed. He is the same yesterday, today, and forever (see Hebrews 13:8). His healing power is available today for you also.

Nahum 1:7 says, *The Lord is good, a stronghold in the day of trouble; and He knows those who trust [take refuge] in Him.*

If you are suffering today, if there is something wrong in your body, I want you to know there is still hope in Jesus.

How I Used the Scriptures to be Healed

The Word of God saved my life. Every day I would read many scriptures.

Proverbs 4:20-22 says, *My son, give attention to my words; incline your ear to my sayings. Do not let them depart from your eyes; keep them in the midst of your heart; for they are life to those who find them, and health to all their flesh.*

To this day, I never leave my home without reading healing scriptures. I know them by heart, but I still look them up and read them. It does something for me.

During my morning quiet time I look at healing scriptures. I don't let them depart from my eyes, keeping them in the midst of my heart, because they have been life and health to me.

The thing I want you to understand is what helped me the most, an unshakable confidence in the Word of God. I knew that if I wasn't getting better it was not God's fault, because God's Word doesn't fail.

You need to make this same decision. Some people get bitter at God when something comes against them, or they don't get well. God is not your enemy! He will keep you alive. It is the devil who wants to destroy you (see John 10:10). Don't get bitter or angry at God. Fight the devil. God wants you well.

You CAN have life abundantly if you want to, but you have to know that it is God's will for you to be healed. Some people who have not studied what the Bible says about healing do not believe it is God's will for them to be healed. They think they must suffer for Jesus. They think that God is teaching them a lesson.

God does not teach His children lessons by making them sick. You don't teach your child a lesson by pushing him in front of a car! God is a loving Father who wants His children well and happy.

One of the scriptures that I read every day was Jeremiah 30:17: *I will restore health to you, and heal you of your wounds*.

There were times I felt as if I was going through a dark tunnel. There seemed to be no end to it, and yet I still confessed, "I am healed."

When anybody would ask me how I felt, I never confessed that I felt bad. I said, "I am blessed of the Lord." I did not tell a lie.

Confession did not seem to work for me for quite a while, but it finally did work! I began to see a faint ray of light. What a wonderful day it was when I saw the bright light of God's healing power!

If you are believing God for something, watch what comes out of your mouth. Keep on confessing the Word of God, and God will honor His Word.

I want you to believe that there is hope in Jesus. I am a person who has been healed of cancer. I am not anybody special. I am one of God's children just like you are. God wants to help you. He wants you to live. He wants you to live a long, healthy, productive life. But your healing doesn't just automatically happen. You must fight your sickness with God's Word and your faith.

Doctors say it is a well-known fact that a feisty person, a fighter, can overcome disease and sickness better than a passive person. There is something in the immune system that goes to work for you when you become a fighter.

Make up your mind that you do not want to die. Plead your case with God. If you have any unforgiveness in your heart, if you have anything in your life that is not pleasing to God, turn away from it. Release it to Jesus. Give your case to God, *casting all your care upon Him, for He cares for you* (1 Peter 5:7).

Now I Want to Pray a Healing Prayer for You

First of all, if you have never given your life to Jesus Christ, you need to be saved. Romans 10:9,10 says, *If you confess with your mouth the Lord Jesus and believe in your heart that God has raised Him from the dead, you will be saved. For with the heart one believes to righteousness, and with the mouth confession is made to salvation.* Give Jesus lordship of your life. Repent of your sins and confess Him as your Lord and Savior and as your Healer. Then you can have confidence to believe God for your complete healing.

Prayer

O God, our Father, Your Word says that You are a very present help in the time of need. I come to You now on behalf of this person who is suffering with cancer, or some other serious disease. Father, I ask You, in the Name of Jesus Christ of Nazareth, to touch and heal them.

Distance is no problem for You, God. As I pray, You are there with them, even as close as the very breath they breathe. So I am asking You to touch their body and heal them.

Now, you foul disease called cancer, I speak to you. Go from this body in the Name of Jesus! I command you, cancerous cells, to wither and die at the roots in the Name of Jesus! Devil, I bind your power in this person's life, and I command healing to come to them now, in the Name of Jesus!

Father, I ask You to replace with new

cells those that have been damaged by cancer or any other disease. God, You can do that, because what is impossible with man is possible with You. You are a God who cares, and we believe You will do it just because we have asked. You love us that much.

Father, may strength and wholeness come into this person's body this very day. Thank You, Lord, for doing it.

I thank You, Jesus, that we will hear good reports from people who have been healed because they held fast to their confession of faith without wavering, because You are faithful who promised. Thank You, Father, in Jesus' Name, Amen.

C H A P T E R   2

Healing Scriptures

One of the most important things that helped me to be healed was the unshakable confidence I had in the Word of God. Many people have asked me for a list of the healing scriptures I used. There are many, but I want to give you the scriptures that helped me most. I still read them every day to build and sustain my faith.

Daily reading of these healing promises was the key to my healing. Use them as part of your daily confession. I believe they will help you in your battle to overcome every symptom and every lie of the enemy.

EXODUS 15:26
Obey God's Word and be healed.
If you diligently heed the voice of the Lord your God and do what is right in His sight, give ear to His commandments and keep all His statutes, I will put none of the diseases on you which I have

brought on the Egyptians [in the permissive sense].
For I am the Lord who heals you.

Are you doing what is right in God's sight?
Are you giving attention to His commandments
and keeping them?

God's promises are conditional, and there are
some things we must do. Hebrews 11:6 says that
God is a *rewarder of those who diligently seek
Him.* If you are not diligently seeking the Lord,
I encourage you to start today. Read and listen to
God's Word. Seek Him with all your heart. Keep
His commandments and change will take place in
your life.

EXODUS 23:25
Serve the Lord and healing will be yours.
*So you shall serve the Lord your God, and He will
bless your bread and your water. And I will take
sickness away from the midst of you.*

This is another wonderful promise to those who
serve the Lord. He'll bless your food and your
water. When I pray over my food at the table, I
never finish without saying, "Father, I thank You
that You have promised to bless our bread and our
water and to take sickness away from our midst."

DEUTERONOMY 7:15
God takes all sickness away from you.
And the Lord will take away from you all sickness, and will afflict you with none of the terrible diseases of Egypt which you have known, but will lay them on all those who hate you.

Notice, it doesn't say, "I will take away from you part of the sickness or certain kinds of sickness," but I will take away from you ALL sickness. This is a wonderful scripture to lean on when the devil tells you your sickness is too difficult for God to heal. No disease is outside God's healing power. Jesus specializes in hard cases, and He is no respecter of persons. He didn't heal me because my husband was John Osteen. He healed me because He loves me and I am His child. He will heal you because He loves you too.

DEUTERONOMY 28:1-2
Now it shall come to pass, if you diligently obey the voice of the LORD your God, to observe carefully all His commandments which I command you today, that the LORD your God will set you high above all nations of the earth. 2 And all these blessings shall come upon you and overtake you, because you obey the voice of the LORD your God.

Then it lists the blessings and the curses. God tells us to diligently obey and observe carefully His commandments. That is when we receive from him.

DEUTERONOMY 30:19
Choose to live. Be a fighter!
I call heaven and earth as witnesses today against you, that I have set before you life and death, blessing and cursing; therefore choose life, that both you and your descendants may live.

It's so important that you choose to live. You must decide that you want to live. Make up your mind and say, "Devil, take your hands off me. I will not let you destroy me. I will not let you kill me. I will not die an early death, but I will live and declare the works of the Lord." As you fight, you will begin to feel better and better and better.

JOSHUA 21:45
God's Word will not fail.
Not a word failed of any good thing which the Lord had spoken….All came to pass.

This scripture helped me so much! It stayed on my mind day and night. I knew God's Word would come to pass. Not one word would fail.

1 KINGS 8:56b
There has not failed one word of all His good promise, which He promised through His servant Moses.

God would never go back on His word nor lie to His children.

PSALM 89:34
My covenant I will not break, Nor alter the word that has gone out of My lips.

You can always count on God to be found faithful.

PSALM 91:16
You will live a long life.
With long life I will satisfy him, and show him My salvation.

This entire chapter is beautiful, but I particularly love to read the 16th verse. When I was fighting cancer, we drove a certain freeway on our way to Lakewood Church where there are two cemeteries. One is small, only about ten graves. As John and I would drive to the church almost every day, when we passed those cemeteries, we would personalize this verse and say, "With long life He satisfies me and shows me His salvation."

PSALM 103:1-5

One of God's benefits is healing.

Bless the Lord, O my soul; and all that is within me, bless His holy name! Bless the Lord, O my soul, and forget not all His benefits. [And what are God's benefits?] *Who forgives all your iniquities, who heals all your diseases, who redeems your life from destruction, who crowns you with lovingkindness and tender mercies, who satisfies your mouth with good things, so that your youth is renewed like the eagle's.*

PSALM 105:37

He also brought them out with silver and gold, And there was none feeble among His tribes.

This was precious to John and me because we called our children, "Our Tribe".

PSALM 107:20

God's Word is healing.

He sent His word and healed them, and delivered them from their destructions.

Again, you can see how important it is to know the Word and to use it for your health and healing. If it had not been for the Word of God, knowing that God's Word works, that God would never lie, and that He keeps His promises, I would not be alive today.

PSALM 118:17

God wants you to live.

I shall not die, but live, and declare the works of the Lord.

This is another scripture that I quote often. When the doctor said I had only a few weeks to live, I made up my mind that I was going to live and not die.

PROVERBS 4:20-22

The Word of God will save your life.

My son, give attention to my words; incline your ear to my sayings. Do not let them depart from your eyes; keep them in the midst of your heart; For they are life to those who find them, and health to all their flesh.

The reason the Word of God is so important when you're fighting a battle for your health is because in many cases it's the only hope you have. That was so in my case.

Give God's Word first place in your heart because it is life and health to your body.

ISAIAH 41:10-13

Fear not, for I am with you; Be not dismayed, for

I am your God. I will strengthen you, Yes, I will help you, I will uphold you with My righteous right hand.' For I, the LORD your God, will hold your right hand, Saying to you, 'Fear not, I will help you.'

Thank God He holds on to us with His right hand.

ISAIAH 43:25-26
Plead your case to God.
I, even I, am He who blots out your transgressions for My own sake; and I will not remember your sins. Put Me in remembrance; let us contend together; state your case, that you may be acquitted.

Verse 26 in the King James Version says, *Put me in remembrance: let us plead together: declare thou, that thou mayest be justified.* I brought my case to God. I prayed, "Father, I plead my case to You, and I ask You to show me things that have been wrong in my life that I can correct."

I pled guilty to a lot of things, and I changed some things.

Then I reminded Jesus of the prayer of agreement that John and I prayed. "Jesus, I want to thank You that on December 11, 1981, in our bedroom, John and I believed that I received my healing, I have it. I rejoice, Jesus, that I'm healed, that all pain and all soreness will be out of my body. It's gone, in Jesus' Name." God honored His Word. Glory!

"Did it leave?" you ask.

No, it didn't leave all at once. I had a spiritual battle to fight. It was as if I were in a dark tunnel. I could see no light for months and months and months. Even so, I never gave up confessing the Word of God, because I had an unshakable confidence in God's Word. I knew Jesus would not lie to me, and I knew that if I kept on believing, I would receive. And I did!

ISAIAH 53:5

Jesus bore your sins AND your sicknesses.

He was wounded for our transgressions, He was bruised for our iniquities; the chastisement for our peace was upon Him, and by His stripes we are healed.

Did you know that Jesus took not only your sins on the cross but also your sicknesses? He bore in His body anything that causes you heartache, poverty, oppression, depression, pain, or suffering. Jesus took it all. Matthew 8:17 refers to Isaiah's prophecy about Jesus, saying, *He Himself took our infirmities and bore our sicknesses.* If Jesus took your sickness, then there is no need for you to bear it. Give it to Him and say, "Jesus, I give this care and heartache to You. It's too much for me. I give this sickness to You, Lord. And I thank You that by Your stripes I am healed!"

JEREMIAH 1:12
Then the LORD said to me, "You have seen well, for I am ready to perform My word."
He will hasten His Word to perform it.

JEREMIAH 30:17
God will restore your health.
For I will restore health to you and heal you of your wounds.
When I was sick, I would look at two pictures of me in radiant health, one in my wedding dress and one riding a horse on a ranch. They bolstered my faith and helped me keep a positive attitude, especially when I was feeling so sick. I kept looking at those pictures and saying, "Thank You, Father, that You will restore health to me and heal me of my wounds. I thank You that I'll feel like I did when I married at 21. I'll feel like I did when I was 25 riding that horse. I thank You that You will restore health to me, Father." When I started feeling good again, I said, "Father, I thank You

that You have restored health to me." I repeat this often, even now.

HOSEA 4:6
My people are destroyed for lack of knowledge.

If you don't know that healing is for today, then you won't know to pray for it.

JOEL 3:10
You can find strength in God and His Word.
Let the weak say, "I am strong."

When you feel weak, repeat this verse, and it will strengthen you. Regardless of how you feel, say, "I'm strong."

Isaiah 27:5 says, *Let him take hold of My strength.* Just reach up and take hold of the Lord's strength. I've done that so many times! I've reached up and said these three little words, "Jesus, help me." And He has never failed to help me. He'll never fail to help you either.

NAHUM 1:9
Your sickness will leave and not come back again.
Affliction will not rise up a second time.

This scripture has been so meaningful to me since I've been healed, because I intend to stay well!

But, know this: The devil is a tormentor, and he will continue to come against you. In the case of cancer, doctors say if you live five years, you're well. But the devil will try to torment you with doubt and fear. If you have a pain, he'll say, "There it is. Cancer is coming back on you." You have to fight these lying imaginations. Cast them down and make every thought line up with the Word.

This is when you can remind the devil of Nahum 1:9. Say, "Devil, this affliction will not rise up the second time. It will never come on my body again!" And it won't!

MALACHI 3:10
Obey all God's commandments and receive all His blessings.

"Bring all the tithes into the storehouse, that there may be food in My house, and prove Me now in this," says the Lord of hosts, "If I will not open for you the windows of heaven and pour out for you such blessing that there will not be room enough to receive it."

In order to diligently obey the voice of the Lord your God, if you follow His commandments, forgiving others, tithing, obeying His commandments, then God will bless you.

MATTHEW 8:2-3

It is God's will for you to be healed.

This scripture says that when the leper came to Jesus, he said, *Lord, if You are willing, You can make me clean. And Jesus said these simple words, I am willing; be cleansed.*

It is God's will for you to be well. If you do not believe that, you need to change your thinking. It is not God who has made you sick, it's the devil. If you have been angry or bitter with God, say, "Father, I've been wrong because I didn't know it was the devil who made me sick. I've been blaming You, and I'm sorry for it. I release this bitterness to You, Jesus. Forgive me."

It is essential to free your heart of anger and bitterness toward God and anyone else so that your prayers will not be hindered.

MATTHEW 8:17

He Himself took our infirmities, And bore our sicknesses.

Jesus took our sins and sicknesses on the cross so we don't have to bear them.

MATTHEW 18:18

You can take authority over the sickness in your body.

Assuredly, I say to you, whatever you bind on earth will be bound in heaven, and whatever you loose on earth will be loosed in heaven.

You can personalize this verse and read it this way: "Whatever I stop on earth will be stopped in heaven, and whatever I permit and allow on earth will be permitted and allowed in heaven."

If you are having symptoms, you can bind those symptoms here on earth and they will be bound in heaven. Rest assured God will keep His Word.

MATTHEW 18:19

Agree with someone for your healing.

Again I say to you that if two of you agree on earth concerning anything that they ask, it will be done for them by My Father in heaven.

This is such an important scripture! If you are married, have your husband or wife agree with you for the healing of your body. Don't let negative thoughts come between you. Jesus said, "When you agree in prayer, it will be done for you by your Father in heaven." After you have agreed and you've asked God to heal you, look up to heaven and say, "Father, we've done what You've told us to do on earth. Now You take over and perform it in heaven." If you don't have anyone to agree with you, agree with God's Word.

MATTHEW 21:21-22
So Jesus answered and said to them, "Assuredly, I say to you, if you have faith and do not doubt, you will not only do what was done to the fig tree, but also if you say to this mountain, 'Be removed and be cast into the sea,' it will be done. 22 And whatever things you ask in prayer, believing, you will receive."

Saying is important. Words can make us or break us.

MARK 11:22-23
What you say will make a difference.
Have faith in God. For assuredly, I say to you, whoever says to this mountain, "Be removed and be cast into the sea," and does not doubt in his heart, but believes that those things he says will be done, he will have whatever he says.

Do you have a mountain of sickness in your body? Do you have a mountain of financial pressures, marital discord, or emotional hurts? Whatever it is, say to it, "Be removed and be cast into the sea," and it will be done. You can see how important it is to say positive statements. The Bible says we are snared by the words of our mouth (see Proverbs 6:2). So watch what you say. Confess, "I believe I am healed," and you will be.

MARK 11:24
Believe, and you will receive.
Therefore I say to you, whatever things you ask when you pray, believe that you receive them, and you will have them.

The day after I came home from the hospital, my husband John and I prayed the prayer of agreement and put my case in the hands of the Lord. As far as I'm concerned, that day, December 11, 1981, my healing began. My body didn't feel healed. In fact, I felt terrible and I looked terrible. But I knew if I gave in to the way I felt, I wouldn't live. I felt like I was going to die so many times! But I fought and I stood firm, and I kept reminding God of His promises in His Word. And I was healed!

MARK 16:17-18
Have someone lay hands on you for healing.
And these signs shall follow those who believe… they will lay hands on the sick, and they will recover.

This is a very effective method Jesus gave for

receiving your healing. Have a minister, or another Christian who believes in healing, lay hands on you and pray for healing. Then believe that you will recover from that time forth.

LUKE 10:19

Behold, I give you the authority to trample on serpents and scorpions, and over all the power of the enemy, and nothing shall by any means hurt you.

JOHN 9:31

Worship God.

If anyone is a worshiper of God and does His will, He hears him.

It is important to worship God. Maybe you've not been used to worshiping God in your church. If not, you can worship Him right now. Just raise your hands and say, "O Jesus, I love You and I worship You. I come before You today, thanking You that Your Word hasn't changed." Worship will make you feel good.

After I read John 9:31, I read John 10:10.

JOHN 10:10

The devil wants to kill you; God wants to heal you.

The thief does not come except to steal, and to kill, and to destroy. I have come that [you] may have life, and that [you] may have it more abundantly.

This is a scripture I quote daily. I read the others, and I don't let them depart from my eyes. But John 10:10 is one that I read aloud every day. I combine John 9:31 and John 10:10, and say, "Devil, you are not going to steal my health. You have not stolen my health, and you will not steal it. You will not kill me, and you will never destroy me, because I am a worshiper of God. I do His will, and He hears me. Jesus has come that I may have life, and have it more abundantly."

ROMANS 4:19-21

And not being weak in faith, he (Abraham) did not consider his own body, already dead (since he was about a hundred years old), and the deadness of Sarah's womb. 20 He did not waver at the promise of God through unbelief, but was strengthened in faith, giving glory to God, 21 and being fully convinced that what He had promised He was also able to perform.

I'm fully convinced that God's Word does not lie.

ROMANS 8:11

The Spirit of Life is making your body alive.

He who raised Christ from the dead will also give life to your mortal bodies through His Spirit who dwells in you.

This verse is so good! The same Spirit that dwelt in Jesus and caused Him to be raised from the dead dwells in me and in you. He is quickening your mortal body, making it alive and vibrant with health. Glory be to the Father!

2 CORINTHIANS 1:20

God is for you.

For all the promises of God in Him are Yes, and in Him Amen, to the glory of God through us.

If you do not know the Word of God, you need to learn it. Many people suffer and die needlessly because they do not know what the Word of God says about healing.

If you're a baby Christian, God will honor that. Don't condemn yourself if you don't know the Word. Just get in the Bible and seek the Lord, and He will show Himself strong on your behalf. If you are in a church where you are not getting good teaching, I would suggest that you go someplace where you can hear the Word of God taught. It may someday keep you alive, as it did in my case.

2 CORINTHIANS 10:4-5
Cast down thoughts and imaginations that don't line up with the Word of God.
For the weapons of our warfare are not carnal, but mighty through God to the pulling down of strongholds; Casting down imaginations, and every high thing that exalteth itself against the knowledge of God, and bringing into captivity every thought to the obedience of Christ (KJV).

When I was sick, I had to cast down imaginations concerning symptoms, and you will, too. Make your thoughts obey you. Bring them into captivity to the obedience of Christ.

Say, "Thoughts, line up with the Word of God that says by the stripes of Jesus I am healed. Thoughts, line up with God's Word that says whatever I ask I receive of Him because I keep His commandments and do those things that are pleasing in His sight. Thoughts, line up with God's Word, in Jesus' Name." And, praise God, it will come to pass!

GALATIANS 3:13-14
You are redeemed from the curse.
Christ has redeemed us from the curse of the law,

having become a curse for us (for it is written, "Cursed is everyone who hangs on a tree"), that the blessing of Abraham might come upon the Gentiles in Christ Jesus.

What was the curse of the law? It was sin, sickness, and poverty. Jesus came into the world and gave himself willingly to die in your place on the cross, redeeming you from the curse. He took the curse of sin, sickness, and poverty upon himself so you wouldn't have to bear it. Thus, He made it possible for you to have the blessings of Abraham, forgiveness, divine health, and provision for your material needs. Praise the Lord!

EPHESIANS 6:10-13
Be strong in the Lord's power. Put on His armor to fight for your healing.
Finally, my brethren, be strong in the Lord and in the power of His might. Put on the whole armor of God, that you may be able to stand against the wiles of the devil. For we do not wrestle against flesh and blood, but against principalities, against powers, against the rulers of darkness of this age, against spiritual hosts of wickedness in the heavenly places. Therefore take up the whole armor of God, that you may be able to withstand in

the evil day, and having done all, to stand.

Verses 14-17 continue: *Stand therefore, having girded your waist with truth, having put on the breastplate of righteousness, and having shod your feet with the preparation of the gospel of peace; above all, taking the shield of faith with which you will be able to quench all the fiery darts of the wicked one. And take the helmet of salvation, and the sword of the Spirit, which is the word of God.*

You need the whole armor of God every day. Resist the devil each day by saying, "Devil, take your hands off me and off my body in Jesus' Name." Then remind your body to line up with the Word of God. It will work!

PHILIPPIANS 2:13

God's will, healing, is working in you.

For it is God who works in you both to will and to do for His good pleasure.

This verse has sustained me in many dark hours. When I'm driving my car or out for a walk, it just rolls out, over and over. I say, "God, You said that You are working in me. You are working in my body both to will and to do for Your good pleasure. Father,

You are working in my mind, renewing it. My health is Your good pleasure."

2 TIMOTHY 1:7
Fear is not of God.
For God has not given us a spirit of fear, but of power and of love and of a sound mind.

I had never been a fearful person. But when cancer tried to attach itself to my body, I had to fight fear.

Now you may think that seems strange, coming from a pastor's wife, and from a Holy Spirit-filled Christian. I don't try to justify it or reason it out. I'm just telling you how it was with me so it might help you.

I'm a human being, and the same things come against me that come against anybody else. So I had to fight fear. And I did it with verses like 2 Timothy 1:7.

I would say, "Father, You haven't given me the spirit of fear, but of power and of love and of a sound mind. This fear is not of You, God. It's of the devil. So I'm commanding it to leave now, in Jesus' Name."

I set a date, September 6, as the day I believed I would be free of the torment of fear. I said, "From this day, I shall have no more fear. It's gone, in Jesus' Name."

If fear is coming against you, rebuke it. Say, "On this day, the day I am reading these words, I'm getting rid of fear. Fear, release me in Jesus' Name. You have no right to torment a child of God. I am full of His peace and love. Now, I cast all of my care upon You, Father, because I know You care for me. And I thank You that I am free from fear." Fear may come, but faith over rules it.

HEBREWS 4:12
For the word of God is living and powerful, and sharper than any two-edged sword, piercing even to the division of soul and spirit, and of joints and marrow, and is a discerner of the thoughts and intents of the heart.
(Soul, spirit, joints, marrow, thoughts and heart. Pretty powerful!)

HEBREWS 10:23
You will not waver in your faith (or heart).
Let us hold fast the confession of our hope without wavering, for He who promised is faithful.

This verse has been so important to me! As I mentioned before, I wavered many times. Of course, it was in my mind, my thoughts, not in my heart! Those accusations that come against you in your mind are from the evil one. The devil is the one who is the accuser of the brethren (see Revelation 12:10). When he tells you anything, believe just the opposite, and you'll have the truth. I learned not to condemn myself any more. I would say, "I thank You, Father, that I am holding fast to my confession without wavering. I don't waver in my spirit man because I know Your Word works."

This will help you, too. If you feel like you are wavering, remember this: you can have doubt in your head but still have faith in your heart.

HEBREWS 10:25
...not forsaking the assembling of ourselves together, as is the manner of some, but exhorting one another.

Church is so important because you hear the Word of God taught, you have fellowship with others, and bring encouragement and get encouragement.

HEBREWS 10:35
You can have confidence in God and His Word.
Therefore do not cast away your confidence,

which has great reward.
Put your confidence in the Lord Jesus Christ and His Word no matter what happens. He is your hope. God will surely reward your trust in Him!

HEBREWS 11:11
By faith Sarah herself also received strength to conceive seed, and she bore a child[a] when she was past the age, because she judged Him faithful who had promised.

HEBREWS 13:8
Jesus Christ has never changed. What He did in the Bible, He will do for you today.
Jesus Christ is the same yesterday, today, and forever.

My husband and I knew so little about healing when our daughter Lisa was born with cerebral palsy and brain damage. John was pastoring a denominational church, and we hadn't been taught about healing.

John and I began to read the four Gospels, Matthew, Mark, Luke, and John, where it tells about the miraculous healings Jesus did and the wonderful things He said.

Then we got over into Hebrews where it said Jesus didn't change. So we prayed, in just the simplest way we knew how, "Jesus, Your Word says You haven't changed. Here we are faced with a little child that has cerebral palsy and brain damage. Father, if You don't change, then You are still the same now. You can touch our little girl and make her whole. Would you touch her and heal her?"

You know, Jesus did just that. Lisa is a perfectly normal adult now, a beautiful young lady. She is strong in the Lord and the power of His might. And she has been such a blessing to us. Jesus hasn't changed. His desire for you is that you be well.

JAMES 1:5
If any of you lacks wisdom, let him ask of God, who gives to all liberally and without reproach, and it will be given to him.

JAMES 3:17
But the wisdom that is from above is first pure, then peaceable, gentle, willing to yield, full of mercy and good fruits, without partiality and without hypocrisy.

JAMES 4:7-8
Therefore submit to God. Resist the devil and he will flee from you. Draw near to God and He will draw near to you.

JAMES 5:14-15

Be anointed with oil by a Christian who believes in healing.

Is anyone among you sick? Let him call for the elders of the church, and let them pray over him, anointing him with oil in the name of the Lord. And the prayer of faith will save the sick, and the Lord will raise him up. And if he has committed sins, he will be forgiven.

I encourage you to call the elders of the church and have them anoint you with oil and pray for you in the name of the Lord. God says the prayer of faith will save the sick.

If you don't have elders who know how to pray the prayer of faith, then find someone who does know how and have them anoint you with oil. Then believe that God will keep His Word, and the Lord will raise you up.

1 PETER 2:24

Jesus has already paid the price for your healing.

Who Himself bore our sins in His own body on the tree, that we, having died to sins, might live for righteousness, by whose stripes you were healed.

Isaiah said, "By His stripes we are healed." Peter,

by revelation of the Holy Spirit, looked back to Isaiah 53:5, and said, "By whose stripes you were healed." Your healing has already been bought and paid for by Jesus himself!

1 PETER 5:7-9
Casting all your care upon Him, for He cares for you. Be sober, be vigilant; because[a] your adversary the devil walks about like a roaring lion, seeking whom he may devour. Resist him, steadfast in the faith.

1 PETER 5:14-15
Be confident in your prayers.
Now this is the confidence that we have in Him, that if we ask anything according to His will, He hears us. And if we know that He hears us, whatever we ask, we know that we have the petitions that we have asked of Him.

How can you pray and ask God for healing in confidence if you don't know that it is His will for you to be healed? You can't! You've learned in the world that if you get sick, you must suffer. And if you're lucky, you might get well. Now you must renew your mind with healing scriptures.

Whatever your need is, find the promise you

need in the Word of God, then ask according to His will. God's will is His Word. When you find a promise for your need, and pray that promise, you will have the confidence that He will hear and answer your prayer.

1 JOHN 3:21-22
God answers the prayers of those who keep His commandments.
Beloved, if our heart does not condemn us, we have confidence toward God. And whatever we ask we receive from Him, because we keep His commandments and do those things that are pleasing in His sight.

If you are not receiving what you need from God, examine yourself. See if you are keeping His commandments and doing those things that are pleasing in His sight.

3 JOHN 2
God's highest wish is for you to be well.
Beloved, I wish above all things that thou mayest prosper and be in health, even as thy soul prospereth (KJV).

Do you know how your soul will prosper? By putting the Word of God in it. Then you will know how to stay in good health. The Lord wants you to walk in divine health. And you can do that by getting the Word of God into your heart. Then when sickness tries to come upon you, you'll be prepared to stand against it.

REVELATION 12:11
Give testimony of your healing.
And they overcame him by the blood of the Lamb and by the word of their testimony.

When God heals you and you recover and are able to testify, do it. The Lord wants you to give glory to Him for what He has done for you.

If you haven't lived for God in the past, He has had mercy on you. Because of His love for you, He touched and healed you. Now, don't go back into the world, but commit yourself completely to Jesus. Serve Him one hundred percent all of your days.

God doesn't heal you to go back into the world. He heals you to set you apart. You're His chosen vessel for Him to live in and to use.

C H A P T E R   3

Physicians' Statements of My Diagnosis and Healing

Dr. Reginald B. Cherry reports:
No hint of disease now present.

To help you understand the magnitude of Dodie Osteen's healing, I want to point out that liver cancer is one of the most treacherous cancers we face in medicine. Because the cancer is in a part of the body that has a high blood supply, a very rich source of nutrients feeds the cancer. In the natural, medical sense, patients live very, very short lifespans once a diagnosis of liver cancer is made. Generally, the weight and energy losses are steady and progressive. And after just a few weeks, six to seven months at the most, the majority of patients succumb to the illness.

In late November 1981, Mrs. Dodie Osteen checked into St. Luke's Hospital at the Texas Medical Center in Houston, Texas, for what she felt would be some routine tests. Her complaint at the time of admission was a history of a mild fever and an episode of right upper quadrant abdominal pain.

Mrs. Osteen's initial physical examination revealed no underlying abnormality. Her blood pressure and skin color were normal. Her heart, lungs, and abdominal examinations were all within normal limits. It was beginning to appear that the mild fever and episodes of upper abdominal pain really weren't anything serious, maybe just a "bug" going around.

The physicians, however, felt an uneasiness. Somehow things just didn't add up. Some of medicine's most sophisticated tests were then ordered. It was after the first of these tests that the first hint of a problem turned up.

The diagnosis was consistent: Cancer!

An abdominal sonogram was performed in which sound waves passed into the abdomen. At first, all images of the pancreas, kidneys, and uterus were normal. Then the radiologist saw the ominous picture. Something was wrong in the liver. There was a mass occupying the right lobe of the liver.

An abdominal C.T. scan, a sophisticated form of X-ray, was ordered, and the results were unequivocal: "large lesion right liver lobe, 2 small lesions left lobe." The scan had the characteristic picture of cancer, but the doctors wanted to be certain. Was it an abscess, possibly caused by an amoeba or a parasite? They had to go into the liver: a biopsy was performed. Special tests were then done for parasites and other organisms, including blood tests, cultures, smears, and stains. All proved negative.

It had to be cancer, and to confirm it, cells were examined by the pathologists. St. Luke's pathologists examined the slides, which were then sent to M.D. Anderson Hospital, a world renowned institution dealing exclusively with the diagnosis and treatment of cancer, also located in the Texas Medical Center. The diagnosis was consistent: "metastatic adenocarcinoma of the liver."

Where, then, was the origin of the cancer? This question remained undetermined. All tests of other organ systems were completely normal.

Mrs. Osteen was informed of the diagnosis. The cancer was classified medically as being incurable. Medicine had reached the end. The sophisticated tests revealed the problem, but the technology of modern medicine could offer little more. Chemotherapy could offer little with this type of cancer. There was no cure. Mrs. Osteen was sent home to die. No medical treatment was given.

Many years have now passed. I have examined Mrs. Osteen on several occasions since that bleak day in 1981. She is now the picture of health. Her physical examination and blood tests are all normal. She is a busy woman, full of energy, and free of any pain. She exercises daily. There is absolutely no hint of disease in her body.

You might well ask, "What happened to Dodie Osteen?"

The answer is simple. She was healed, not in the traditional medical sense, but supernaturally, in answer to prayer. I thank God for the healing Dodie Osteen has experienced. God touched her in a special way. We're discovering some tremendous things in medicine today, especially about how attitude affects healing. We're learning now that a person's positive attitude in fighting and refusing to accept illness can literally change white blood cell counts in the body. It can actually activate a defense the body naturally has against disease, and against cancer in particular.

A Miracle is Obvious

The natural inclination of the human mind is to say, "The doctors missed the diagnosis. It wasn't really cancer."

If only one doctor had followed this case, yes maybe the diagnosis could be an error. Mistakes are made. This case, however, was different. It was reviewed by numerous pathologists, radiologists, and internists, all experts in cancer diagnosis and treatment. Their opinions were all the same: "a typical picture of metastatic adenocarcinoma of the liver." The diagnosis was obvious to them. Mrs. Osteen had cancer. It has now, however, become equally obvious that Mrs. Osteen has been healed of cancer.

The miracle of supernatural healing is real. As a physician, I practice with the most sophisticated tools known to man. However, medicine frequently reaches its end, with nothing further to offer a patient. Every human being, at one time or another, will need a miracle from God...maybe in the area of healing or with some other need. I see miracles, the supernatural healings of God, almost daily in my practice.

Why don't I see or hear of more miracles like Dodie Osteen's?

The answer is straightforward. God manifests Himself to us in the area in which we are willing to believe Him. If a person believes God for salvation and eternal life, God will manifest Himself in this way. Dodie Osteen believed God for her healing, and God manifested himself to her in this way. Through His mercy and love, God touched her body and supernaturally healed her. God is no respecter of persons. He is willing to heal anyone if they will only believe.

Dodie Osteen's story is a dramatic and thrilling one. After going through this ordeal, I told Pastor and Mrs. Osteen that, considering the kind of cancer she had, they could never fully appreciate the magnitude of her healing. As a medical doctor, I am, of course, thankful for the great sophistication of modern medicine. But in the end, it is God who heals. Physicians only treat.

Reginald B. Cherry, MD

Dr. Richard W. Walker, Jr. reports:
No Trace of Cancer

My family and I have attended Lakewood Church in Houston, Texas, since 1979. Over the years, my wife and I have gotten to know the pastor and his wife, John and Dodie Osteen, quite well. Dodie eventually became one of my patients.

Prior to Pastor Osteen's announcement to the church of Dodie's illness, I mentioned to my wife privately that the pastor's wife didn't appear to be well. She walked slowly and unsteadily as she approached the pulpit. Her voice was unsteady, and her skin was sallow. She didn't speak with the boldness and joy she once did.

About three weeks later, the pastor came to the church without Mrs. Osteen. My wife and I knew something was wrong. The pastor entered the pulpit with fatigue showing in his voice and face, and announced that his wife was seriously ill and asked us to pray for her continuously...which we did.

I saw Mrs. Osteen for the first time as a patient on July 5, 1985. By this time, she was well recovered from her battle with cancer. She came because she had known for quite some time that she had a fibroid tumor on her womb (uterus).

A fibroid tumor of the womb is generally a benign tumor of the muscle of the wall of the uterus. This fibroid tumor had been present for years and was originally diagnosed by her former gynecologist. Because of its size, nothing needed to be done then. However, Mrs. Osteen began experiencing symptoms related to the fibroid tumor.

My examination revealed a uterine fibroid tumor, which I described as follows: "Uterus: anteroverted with a golf ball-sized mass on the posterior left fundus." This meant there was a mass on the back wall of the uterus, measuring approximately five centimeters in diameter.

I sent for the records of Mrs. Osteen's ultrasound report done several days prior to this office visit. The report substantiated my findings. It read:

"Opinion: Enlargement of the uterus, fibroids versus neoplasm [other tumors]. Hepatic [liver] mass...benign or malignant." This report described the presence of two findings, one in the womb, the other in the liver.

No Tumor Found

Although Mrs. Osteen was spiritually at peace, she was struggling in her mind as to whether she should have surgery to remove the uterus with the fibroid tumor. She finally resolved that a hysterectomy needed to be performed.

An examination, performed while Mrs. Osteen was under anesthesia immediately before surgery, demonstrated she had a golf ball-sized tumor. After surgery, the pathological report revealed no tumor was found in the uterus!

One might ask at this point, if God healed Dodie of cancer earlier, why didn't He also remove the fibroid tumor at the same time? I don't know! The answer to this question is one that only the great I AM can answer. However, had I not documented the latter event, I would never have been able to confirm God's healing of Dodie Osteen. He blessed me to be a part of her miracle.

During the course of my treatment of Mrs. Osteen since July 5, 1985, I have made a thorough examination of her on several occasions, and can state that she is now in perfect health. As I stated, I observed her when she was ill with cancer. I read her medical records and test results by other physicians which indicated "metastatic adenocarcinoma [cancer] of the liver."

I know that after the diagnosis of liver cancer was made, no further medical treatment was administered. Seeing Dodie Osteen after her cancer and treating her for her uterine tumor, I can categorically state that many years later there is no trace of any disease. Indeed, she is now a normal, strong, healthy woman.

Richard W. Walker, Jr., MD was in private practice in obstetrics and gynecology in Clear Lake, Texas.

The late D. L. Moore, MD:
The diagnosis was well established.

Dear Pastor Osteen,

You will recall I helped you pick your primary physician in Houston who is a highly regarded specialist who graduated from Harvard Medical School. I knew his professional capabilities, his spirit, as well as his Christian outlook on life. As he hospitalized Dodie, ran tests and performed examinations at St. Luke's Hospital, I received frequent reports. When he firmed up his diagnosis, I had a chance to review all of Dodie's reports and X-rays. I quote his conclusions in the last part of his own letter to me:

Physicians' Statements

"Since the presence of mesothelial cells was puzzling and I thought unlikely, I asked for the slides to be reviewed by other members of the pathology department at St. Luke's Hospital, and also by the pathologists at the M. D. Anderson Hospital. On review, it was the consensus of the pathologists, that indeed these cells were not mesothelial cells, but were quite characteristic of adenocarcinoma. The diagnosis therefore seemed well established that the so-called cyst in actuality is necrotic tumor. The original CT scan of the liver showed this one large mass almost completely replacing the right lobe of the liver and two much smaller masses in the left lobe of the liver.

Doctor and Mrs. Osteen were both informed of this diagnosis. They elected to be discharged from the hospital for reflection and prayer for healing, and Mrs. Osteen was discharged."

The diagnosis was well established in my opinion. As you know, Dodie slowly but surely returned to her visible health I had known and observed prior to her illness. Now, after several years, she has remained well. When I examine her countenance and vitality now, I can come to one conclusion only, that Dodie has been healed miraculously by prayers. To me there can be only one conclusion: God answered your prayers and healed her.

I must tell you that knowing all the players and having seen all the tests and X-rays has made a tremendous impact on me. It is one thing to read about miracles, but it is another to sit by and watch one happen.

Sincerely and with wishes for your continued happiness and impact on others, I remain devotedly yours,

The late **D. L. Moore, MD**
Texas

CHAPTER 4

Frequently Asked Questions

People ask me all the time how I am doing, and I am so thankful to say that the Lord Jesus has blessed me in abundance. After more than twenty years, I am still strong and healthy, and I plan to stay that way!

In 1981, when I was diagnosed with metastatic cancer of the liver, with just a few weeks to live, it was a very dark and dismal day for me and for John and our family. The day after I left the hospital, when John and I laid on our faces on the floor of our bedroom, and he commanded the cancer in my body to wither and die, just like Jesus did the fig tree in the spirit realm, the roots of the cancer died. It did not feel like it had died, but Psalm 56:9 says, *The day that we pray, the tide of the battle turns* (TLB).

People have asked me in the past about several things, and I thought it might help if I answered some of the questions. They want to know if I went on a special diet or took mega doses of vitamins.

I had been a healthy eater for years before I got sick, so I did not really change my eating habits. Through the years I have taken daily vitamins. Some doctors recommend mega vitamins, so it is just up to the individual.

I am often asked how long I prayed each day. That is a question that tormented me. I had heard someone say that we should pray six hours a day, and I didn't do that, so I got under condemnation that I wasn't pleasing God. I realized that the devil was coming against me with tormenting accusations, and that I prayed continually during the day. When I drove the car I prayed, when I walked to the mailbox I prayed, and when I cooked I prayed. My meditations were on the Lord Jesus, day and night.

People wonder how long I had pain. This is a question that I do not like to answer, because no two cases are alike. I found out that when I was fighting a battle and called to pray for other people on the phone, as they talked about their symptoms, the devil would try to put the same symptoms on me. People have different thresholds of pain, and it is not good to compare cases.

I mentioned in my book that the doctor could not find a primary tumor, so no chemotherapy was advised. We are not against chemotherapy, or radiation, or doctors or medicine. We want people to get well any way they can. Each person has to "let the peace of God rule in their heart" (see Colossians 3:15). When Jesus raised Lazarus from the dead, He told the disciples to roll away the stone. He told them to do what they could do, and He would do what they couldn't do. They moved and He moved. God wants you to do what you can do and trust Him for what you can't do.

There are many different ways of healing, but only one Healer, and His name is Jesus. He wants His children well. And I trust that this book will be a means of bringing hope to your heart and to always know that He will never change.